Resistance Rising: Genetics, Evolution, and the Future of Infectious Diseases

Brian Pollo

Published by Sandiwà Press, 2025.

RESISTANCE RISING: GENETICS, EVOLUTION, AND THE FUTURE OF INFECTIOUS DISEASES

First edition. September 18, 2025.

ISBN: 979-8232778415

Written by Brian Pollo.

Also by Brian Pollo

Hiyang: Pilipinong Pananaw ng Parmakohenetika
Hiyang: Pilipinong Pananaw ng Parmakohenetika
Salinlunas: Natural Products & Pharmacognosy
Salinlunas: Natural Products & Pharmacognosy
Currents of Protection
Currents of Protection
Resistance Rising: Genetics, Evolution, and the Future of Infectious Diseases
Resistance Rising: Genetics, Evolution, and the Future of Infectious Diseases
Phonies: Authenticity Performance Fakery
Phonies: Authenticity Performance Fakery
Biographies in Blood: The Making of Medical Modernity and Asian Medical Innovations

Watch for more at https://sites.google.com/view/brian-pollo/home.

Table of Contents

For

MD-PhD (molecular medicine)

Batch 6 of the

University of the Philippines

College of Medicine

"Nothing in biology makes sense except in the light of evolution."

Theodosius Dobzhansky

Summary

This book expounds on genetic and evolutionary explanations that inform insights regarding antimicrobial resistance and infectious diseases. Resistance is a problem threatening the revolutionary contributions of antimicrobials to humanity. The emergence and establishment of antimicrobial resistance is facilitated by (*i*) the spread of antimicrobial resistance genes (which may be harbored in higher-order biological units, *e.g.*,, mobile genetic elements, bacterial communities, etc.), but also by (*ii*) the human- mediated spread of ecotoxic agents (particularly antimicrobials) which accelerate evolutionary rates both through stress induction and selection. An outdated conception of antimicrobials is a contributor to this environmental pollution and proliferation of resistant biological units. Keeping in mind that humans and microbes have a long coevolutionary history, perhaps we ought to drive the evolution of less virulent microbes rather than engage in an unwinnable evolutionary arms race. Lastly, recurring lessons for the future suggest that (*i*) systems/networks also exhibit 'illness', and that (*ii*) the evolutionary consequences of humanity ought to be recognized.

0. Preface

If we wish to continue using antimicrobials to benefit our health, we need to address antimicrobial resistance. The primary motivation in trying to address antimicrobial resistance is the fear that the utility of antimicrobials would eventually be diminished, to the point where it is more probable that an antimicrobial would be ineffective for a particular clinical use. Important definitions to clarify in the discussion of antimicrobial resistance are those of 'resistance' and 'resistance genes'.

In line with the realization that the major motivation for human antimicrobial use (*i.e.,* treatment of infections) is affected by both microbe and host factors, section 2 of this book will be microbe-centric, section 3 will be host- (or human-), while section 4 will look at their shared experience (i.e., host-microbe coevolution with attendant discussion of virulence). The emergence and spread of resistance genes will be described in section 2 concomitant with an exposition on microbial genetic diversity. Then, historical/evolutionary perspectives on human antimicrobial use and the origin of antimicrobials will be discussed in sections 3 and 4.

1. Motivation

Before we proceed further, the definition of antimicrobial resistance ought to be clarified first. The term 'antimicrobial' may imply this definition: "agents that kill or inhibit the growth of microorganisms, *i.e.,*, organisms that could not be seen by the naked eye.". Such a definition would therefore exclude infectious agents once they are visible to the naked eye. Also, such a definition would include microscopic non infectious organisms, *e.g.,* tardigrades. Due to these non-useful qualities, this definition of 'antimicrobial' is rejected in this paper. In this book, an antimicrobial is an agent that kills or inhibits the growth of infectious agents. In other words, this paper adopts a definition of 'antimicrobial' akin to that of 'anti-infective'. For the purposes of this paper, antimicrobials include antibiotics (used against bacteria), antivirals (used against viruses), antifungals (used against fungi), antiprotozoals (used against protistan parasites), and anthelmintics (used against helminthic parasites). Also, this paper adopts a definition of 'microbe' akin to that of 'infectious agent'. A microbe therefore is a living agent that exists in a host—not necessarily causing disease. The precise meaning of antimicrobial resistance would depend on the context in which it is used (American Academy of Microbiology, 2010): (*i*) In a clinical paradigm, antimicrobial resistance would refer to the survival of an infectious agent at concentrations that would typically kill other infectious agents (*i.e.,* clinical breakpoints), (*ii*) in a biological paradigm, antimicrobial resistance would refer to the reduced susceptibility of an infectious agent relative to other typical infectious agents (*n.b.*, this definition does not hinge on a preset breakpoint), and (*iii*) in a genomic paradigm, antimicrobial resistance would refer to the presence of genes that contribute to the expression of a phenotype marked by diminished susceptibility to infectious agents. In the present work, antimicrobial resistance is viewed from a broad perspective. Perhaps the biological and genomic definitions most closely approximate the usage of 'antimicrobial resistance' in this mini-review. The inherent of ambiguity of terminology in this present work may be desirable in order to recognize broad themes and patterns that traverse precise reductionist definitions so commonly occurring in human perspectives.

1.1. A gene-based definition of resistance

CLINICAL DEFINITIONS of resistance are based on the minimum inhibitory concentration (MIC). This approach has its greatest utility in ascertaining the likelihood of therapeutic failure in humans. Nevertheless, it has inadequacies in surveilling for low-level increases in resistance (*i.e.,* those that do not register at the inhibitory breakpoint) that may further lead to the development of high-level (hence clinically relevant) resistance. Further disadvantages include the inapplicability of current data for organisms that are not associated with humans, and for antimicrobials not used therapeutically. In themid-1990s, common epidemiological cut-off values for resistance (ECOFFs) were defined by the European Committee on Antimicrobial Susceptibility Testing (EUCAST) as the minimum inhibitory concentration (MIC) value that is the upper limit of the wild-type population of a particular species. ECOFF breakpoints overcomes the disadvantage of limited applicability of clinical definitions. ECOFF breakpoints may be practically used for any microbe-antimicrobial organism. Nevertheless, its primary disadvantage lies in its requirement of analyzing numerous isolates (collected independently) in order to determine a wild-type MIC distribution for a particular microbial species. Further, it merely examines resistance at a species level, and hence has little utility for studying gene level increases in mutation. Genomic definitions of resistance would operationally consist of a pairwise comparison between (*i*) a parental strain and a (*ii*) strain which may be a mutant, or may have acquired antimicrobial resistance by horizontal gene transfer (HGT). Nevertheless, further ecological definitions of resistance genes have been proposed (Martínez et al., 2014). The central premise of this definition is that resistance genes are those that function to protect an organism from an antimicrobial utilized by another organism. Before its implications are further discussed, forms of resistance ought to be described.

Resistance may be (*i*) an ability innate to the microbe to resist an antimicrobial (intrinsic resistance), or (*ii*) an ability obtained through mutation or HGT (acquired resistance). Perhaps the simplest case intrinsic resistance is the absence of the drug target (Blair et al., 2015). The identification of the genes responsible for intrinsic resistance may be informative in the selection of antimicrobials against a particular microbial clade. Liu et al. (2010) performed the identification of genes responsible for intrinsic antibiotic resistance (against β-lactams, aminoglycosides, and fluoroquinolones) found in *Staphylococcus aureus, Pseudomonas aeruginosa,* and *Escherichia coli.* Their methodology involved high-throughput antibiotic susceptibility screening of genome mutant libraries (which, in turn, were generated either through random mutagenesis or targeted insertion). Acquired resistance, on the other hand, may involve the following mechanisms: (*i*) prevention of access to the target (through an impermeable barrier, or through the action of efflux pumps), (*ii*) modification of targets (through target site mutation, or target site protection), or (*iii*) direct interaction with antimicrobials (through hydrolytic degradation, or functional group modification). Whether the genes encoding for these classically recognized types of resistance may now be examined in the light of the ecological definition of a resistance gene.

It may be noted that these resistance mechanisms pertain to individual microbes. Nevertheless, resistance may be a population phenomenon. Population resistance is manifested in bacteria through biofilm formation, in which the bacterial community (*i*) forms in effect a mechanical barrier against antimicrobial access, and (*ii*) undertakes signaling that cause changes (*e.g.,* phenotypic changes) among members of the community (Penesyan, 2015). Indeed, resistance networks are multi-level, and resistance therefore may be viewed through various scales and resolutions (Stokes, 2011). For instance, individual resistance genes may be found in different resistance-conferring genetic transfer units, which in turn occur in resistant organisms that may form communities/populations exhibiting resistance properties.

Genes may be present in an antimicrobial-producing organisms that code for enzymes specifically capable of deactivating the compounds produced by the same organism. Although these are conventionally considered as resistance genes, Martínez et al. (2014) propose that these should be treated as detoxification genes because it does not protect from an antimicrobial produced by a competitor. Via a similar logic, porin genes and multidrug (MDR) efflux pump genes ought not to be classified as resistance genes. Kojima (2013) has suggested that the major porins in *Enterobacteriaceae* (*viz.,* OmpC and OmpF of E. coli) primarily function as nonspecific channels. Further, former evidence suggesting the existence of drug binding sites in these porins now appear to be false (Tran, et al., 2013). Turning now to efflux pumps, their ubiquity suggests origins and function other than to transport antimicrobials specifically. Efflux pumps are ubiquitous and typically did not evolve to confer resistance to antimicrobials currently anthropologically utilized (Piddock, 2006). For instance, AcrAB in E. coli most probably evolved to confer resistance to bile salts. Also, the majority of efflux pumps are MDR efflux pumps that display a wide substrate range. Evidence to MDR efflux pump ubiquity is that in recent years, previously undescribed pumps continue to be reported in literature, *e.g.,* LmrS in *Staphylococcus aureus* (Floyd et al, 2010), MdeA in *Streptococcus mutans*, and KexD in *K. penumoniae* (Kim, et al., 2013).

Although one classically accepted source of antimicrobial resistance genes is the producer of the antimicrobial, it is also accepted that resistance genes could arise (typically from housekeeping genes) in potentially any microbe because the precursors are also found in them. For instance, aminoglycoside and macrolide inactivating enzymes descended from the ancestral proteins Ser/Thr/Tyr protein kinases (Shakya and Wrigh, 2010). In the aftermath of complete sequencing of bacterial genomes, it has now been realized that bacteria possess numerous alternate pathways towards the emergence of resistance. The collection of resistance genes and their precursors, therefore, has now been conceptually termed the resistome. It encompasses both (*i*) conventionally accepted resistance genes, (*ii*) cryptic resistance genes, and (*iii*) precursor genes. Cryptic resistance genes are phenotypically silent, *i.e.,* their presence does not confer resistance because their expression does not reach a sufficient threshold. Precursor genes, on the other hand, have the potential for evolving into a gene capable of conferring resistance.

These ecological clarifications on the definition of resistance genes merely suggest that a definition would have to be based on the contextualization of a gene. For instance, AcrAB in gut bacteria is normal but its presence in other environments (*e.g.,* aquatic bodies) may suggest fecal pollution. Further, the transfer of a gene from an organism found in an environment in which that gene has conferred resistance to an organism that typically causes human disease (*i.e.*, that typically engaged in a pathogenic interaction) represents a decontextualization. Overall, the definition of a resistance gene ought to be primarily based around its probability of being incorporated to an organism that may cause human disease (*i.e.,* a typical pathogen). Baquero and colleagues (2014) proposed 7 resistance readiness condition (RESCon) levels (RESCon 1being the highest risk, while

RESCon 7 being the lowest) based on an ecologically informed definition of resistance genes.

The RESCon levels and other attempts at arriving at a definition of resistance highlight the difficulty in constructing satisfactory resistance definitions free from ambiguity. The difficulty lies in the emergent nature of resistance. There is no strict criterion that delineates resistance genes from any other housekeeping gene. Indeed, resistance genes typically occur through a decontextualization (from evolutionary context, such that housekeeping genes in environmental microbes exhibit resistance functions in human-associated microbes. Our conception of resistance and resistance genes, therefore, ought not to be reductionist; instead, one must realize that the resistance problem may have to be solved by multi- sectoral inter-disciplinary approaches.

1.2. The dwindling antimicrobial drug discovery pipeline

AS AN ADDENDUM, IT may be noted that the problem of antimicrobial resistance is compounded by the dwindling drug discovery pipeline (Coates, 2011). Resistant strains have been found in clinical isolates a few years (and in some cases such as levofloxacin, within the same year, Figure 1) after introduction of antimicrobials in the market. In the future, it is expected that new classes of antibiotics are necessary to maintain the current utility of antibiotics in medicine. Coates (2011) for instance predicts that 40 new classes are needed in the next century. The reason behind this ready appearance of

antimicrobial resistance in clinical settings is rooted in the environmental ubiquity of resistance genes and the mobility of most of these genes. This will be described in further sections.

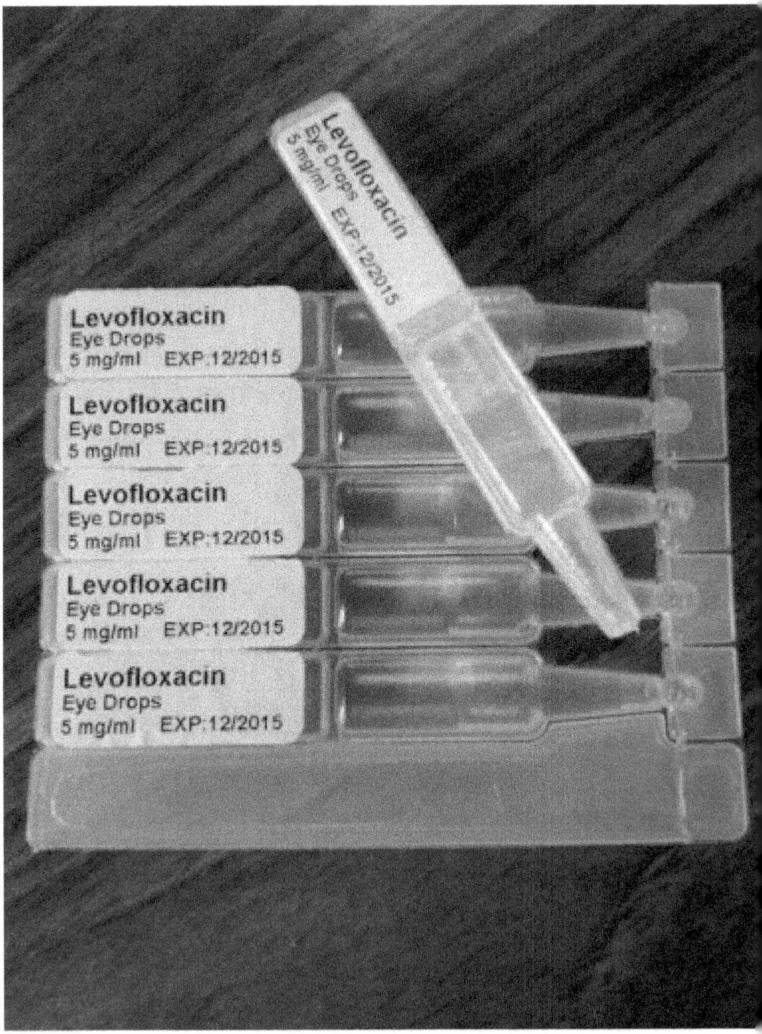

Figure 1. Levofloxacin. Victuallers, CC BY-SA 3.0 <https://creativecommons.org/licenses/by-sa/3.0>, via Wikimedia Commons

2. Microbial evolution of resistance

The evolvability of antimicrobial resistance may be described follows (Falconer, 1981): The change in mean intergenerational value of antimicrobial resistance is the product of (*i*) genetic variance of antimicrobial resistance, and (*ii*) intensity of selection. The capacity of microbial systems for evolution, therefore, may be described by discussing (*i*) sources of genetic novelty (*viz.,* mutation, and other combinatorial processes), and (*ii*) limitations to diversity (*viz.,* selection and drift).

2.1. The emergence of resistance

A KEY MICROBIAL EVOLUTIONARY strategy is its general genome identity fluidity, at least relative to humans. Unlike multicellular organisms that generally have a huge stake in maintaining germline sequences, prokaryotes undergo more novelty-generating processes. Some properties broadly exhibited by microbes are: (*i*) that they possess less stringent controls in the emergence of diversity, (*ii*) that they possess simpler genomes facilitating less lag time in the manifestation of phenotypic effects, and (iii) that they exhibit large population sizes, facilitating more genetic 'trial-and-error' (González-Candelas, 2011).

The sources of genetic variation (i.e., novelty) may be divided into: (*i*) mutation, (*ii*) combinatorial processes (e.g., recombination and amplification), and (*iii*) migration (when there is a spatial component to the distribution of genetic diversity). Mutation and recombination may generate within-population diversity, while migration could introduce diversity in a population if there is a spatial structuring involved (Morgan and Koskella, 2011). Although the frequency of these mechanisms in a population are variable, occurrences are typically 10^{-9} – 10^{-6} for mutation, 10^{-7} – 10^{-3} for recombination, and 10^{-5} – $10^{-2}$for amplification. When it is recognized that large bacterial populations—typically >108 cells/mL in their respective niches—are usually involved, these seemingly infrequent occurrences of novelty may be recognized to be considerable generators of variation. The corollary, however, is that resistant mutants are relatively less frequently generated by reduced population sizes (*e.g.,* when population growth is held in check by immunity or therapy, and when transmission bottlenecks occur in the course of microbial mobility (González-Candelas, 2011).

Further contributors to microbial genetic diversity may now be enumerated (Lederberg, 1998), including those pertaining to (*i*) DNA replication, (*ii*) RNA replication, (*iii*) mutagens, (*iv*) haploidy, and (*v*) phase variation.

DNA replication is typically more error-prone in microbes than in humans. Aside from a 'baseline' incidence of mutation, hypermutability may occur in some instances. For example, some bacteria (termed mutators) that display 10X to 1000X chance of introducing sequence changes in the course of a replication cycle. Hypermutation is largely an effect of defective mismatch repair systems. Hypermutability leads to a heightened probability of generating resistance genes. In the presence of antimicrobials, mutators present and advantage. Thus, mutator strains have been utilized in research to predict the emergence and subsequent selection of resistant variants. Stepanova (2008) utilized a hypermutable *E. coli* nosocomial strain in order to identify a mutation granting additional ceftazidime resistance in CTX M-3 β-lactamase.

In a more specific case, precise replication in bacteria may be turned off in an SOS response (*e.g.,* to injury in the form of DNA damage) leading to hypermutability. The SOS response is triggered essentially by DNA damage. In an SOS response, there is increased expression of error-prone polymerases. For instance, in the case of E. coli, RecA protomers assemble at single-stranded DNA sites, leading to the formation of a RecA filament. This would lead to the autocleavage of LexA, a repressor for the transcription of various regulated genes (*e.g.*, LexA for negative feedback, uvrABC for nucleotide excision repair, recA for homologous recombination, dinA encoding pol II, dinB encoding pol IV, and umuDC encoding pol V). The low-fidelity polymerases have 100X less fidelity than Pol II (PolB). One SOS response trigger is the accumulation of toxic reactive oxygen species as a result of bactericidal antibiotic action. Bactericidal antibiotics, therefore, cause a concomitant increase in microbial genetic diversity apart from their killing action. An illustrative example of this was described in the paper of Da Re, et al. (2009), in that ciprofloxacin treatment induced SOS response, increased expression of error-prone polymerases, cleavage of LexA (a negative repressor of qnrB2, a fluoroquinolone resistance gene, eventually leading to the overexpression of QnrB (a protein that binds to DNA gyrase and protects it from fluoroquinolone action).

RNA replication is error prone too especially in the absence of proofreading capability to examine its fidelity. The concept of a subspecies swarm becomes important when considering biological units (*e.g.*, RNA viruses, especially retroviruses) displaying high mutation rates such that a unit is approximately genotypically different (by at least a nucleotide) with another unit. A viral quasispecies is a cluster or 'cloud' of variants that differ by virtue of mutations, but whose identity revolve around consensus sequences (representing that which provide the greatest fitness).

Microbes are typically capable of existing in the presence of physical and chemical mutagens. While humans take great care to avoid mutagens (*e.g.*, UV, nitrites, polycyclic aromatic hydrocarbons), microbes are capable of existing in conditions where mutagens simultaneously exist. Haploidy may contribute to the ability of microbes to respond to changes in environmental selection pressure. A consequence of haploidy is that there is no delay in expressing genetic factors, thus resulting in a prompt manifestation of amputation. Another contributor to microbial genetic diversity is phase variation. Phase variation is a way for parasites to adaptively change by accessing its genetic archive. Site-specific recombinases may rearrange the parasite such that genes are silenced or unsilenced. Protozoan parasites may be cited for their existence in various phases as they traverse various hosts. The VSG (variant surface glycoprotein) cassettes of trypanosomal parasites may also be cited for their role in the difficulty of developing trypanosomal vaccines.

Classically, resistance evolution is simplistically described as selection of mutations. Vere Hodge, et al. (2011), for instance, maintains that this is the general case, as exemplified by their one principle mechanism for the development of resistance. It has to be highlighted, however, that certain processes apart from mutation and selection are important, particularly in the microbial case. Aside from mutations, combinatorial processes are also major contributors to diversity. Horizontal gene transfer is a particularly important interindividual combinatorial process that could lead to the transmission of resistance. Also, aside from selection, drift is a major limit to diversity that could lead to the predomination of resistance gene in a population. Nevertheless, mutations are major sources of phenotypic changes, especially relative to epigenetic changes or repeat variations (Jansen, 2015).

The emergence of resistance typically occurs through a series of mutations, although it may also occur through a single mutation especially if the mechanism involves the acquisition of a mobile genetic element or efflux protein overexpression. There is a cost of resistance such as when resources are diverted to the production of proteins devoted to resistance mechanisms. This cost may occur because it involves plasmid introduction. Alternatively, the resistance-conferring mutation may affect an essential microbial enzyme. The cost of resistance may be surmounted in compensatory evolution. There is an intuitive sense that compensation is more likely than reversion considering that there are more loci that can restore the fitness cost associated with resistance emergence, while reversion would require, at least in the case of chromosomal mutation, a change of the particular codon involved into its wild type. The mechanisms in the compensation of the fitness cost of antimicrobial resistance may be: (*i*) chromosomal mutation, (*ii*) alteration of expression, or (*iii*) bypass. Chromosomal mutations involve secondary compensatory mutations occurring after the initial resistance-generating mutation. These may occur in the protein affected by the resistance mutations in which case it is intragenic, or it may occur in some other protein, in which case it is intergenic. Once an initial resistance mutation occurs, a secondary stabilizing mutation occurs in order to further increase fitness (compensating for the cost that may have been incurred by the primary mutation. Thus resistance emergence is typically multistep. Also, once resistance emerges, it is not easily reversible.

Another important consideration in the pathways (consisting of a series of mutations) of the emergence of antimicrobial resistance enzymes is interaction of mutations. Epistasis (Figure 2) refers to the non-additive interaction of mutations. Epistatic interactions are especially important because they determine which evolutionary pathways are accessible in the presence of selection. Epistasis is also a key determinant of the evolvability of organisms (particularly their proteins). Sign epistasis (epistatic interactions which may be beneficial or deleterious in particular fitness contexts) may be (i) positive sign epistasis or (ii) negative sign epistasis. In epistasis, and even more importantly in sign epistasis, the sequence and combination of mutational occurrence are of importance. When mutational pathways characterized by fitness in a selective context (*e.g.,* resistance in the presence of antimicrobials) are mapped, a fitness landscape may be generated characterized by mutational trajectories connecting adaptive peaks of different intensities. The topography of this fitness landscape would be heavily dictated by epistasis.

Positive sign epistasis is predicated on the stabilization of protein configuration in the case of combined mutations as opposed to single mutations which may be deleterious. On the other hand, negative sign epistasis (or reciprocal sign epistasis), occurs when mutations that are beneficial individually become deleterious when combined. Novais, et al. (2008) described such a case in which the simultaneous presence of D240G and P167S mutations in CTX-M β-lactamases lead toward a lower efficiency of hydrolyzing ceftazidime than that conferred by each alone. Dellus-Gur (2015) explained an instance of negative sign mutation in which R164S and G238S mutations (which confer TEM-1 β-lactamase activity against 2nd and

3rd generation cephalosporins) induce disorder such that the Asn170 residue (coordinated with the deacylating water molecule) becomes misaligned. In this case, in which the enzyme activity could not be restored by stabilizing mutations, the mutational interaction has led to an evolutionary cul- de-sac.

Although single-nucleotide mutations have traditionally been the mainstay in the human understanding of genetic variation, current knowledge supports the relevance of other mechanisms of genetic variance generation. Apart from the vertical transmission of genes (*i.e.,* parent to offspring), there is horizontal gene transfer (HGT) also referred to as lateral gene transfer (LGT). HGT requires (*i*) a transfer mechanism, and (*ii*) an integration mechanism (Stokes, 2011).

The three major normally occurring transfer mechanisms in bacteria include: (*i*) conjugation in which physical contact between a donor and a recipient cell occurs trough a conjugation pilus (through which genetic material is transferred), (*ii*) transduction in which delivery occurs through phage predation (owing to integration of exogenous host genetic material into a phage genome), and (*iii*) transformation in which there is uptake of exogenous DNA from the environment (Soucy, 2015).

Mobile genetic elements (collectively termed the mobilome) facilitate movement of resistance genes between individual prokaryotes, and these MGEs include: (*i*) integrons (whose structure will be discussed below), (ii) transposons (DNA elements, flanked by repeats, that can move between locations, but could not integrate independently), and (iii) plasmids (circular DNA that may replicate independently of the bacterial chromosome). (Norman, 2009)

The integron is worthy of further discussion. An integron is composed of: (*i*) int, a gene encoding for a site-specific recombinase belonging to the integrase family (*ii*) attI, attC, which are recombination sites, and (*iii*) Pc, promoter (which may or may not be present, and may be multiple, and may also be found internally between gene cassettes). Gene cassettes (including those conferring resistance to antibiotics, disinfectants, and heavy metals) are inserted by intI-mediated recombination at the attI and attC sites. Integrons have conserved sequences upstream of intI and in boundary regions (*i.e.*, flanking cassettes). (Gillings, 2015)

There is such a diversity of genes available to a prokaryote aside from those in its chromosomal DNA, that the supergenome has been used as a collective term for all the genes accessible to a prokaryote (including those in its chromosome, and those in its environment (Norman, 2009). The enrichment of the supergenome with resistance genes and MGEs has been associated by anthropogenic antimicrobial use. The occurrence of HGT is balanced by forward drivers, such as the need for phenotypic novelty in the face of selection pressure (e.g., environmental antimicrobials, and backward drivers, such as (i) the needfor genotypic integrity (*e.g.*, phage resistance, and barriers to transposon incorporation), and (ii) the cost of MGEs and selfish genetic elements (*e.g.,* plasmids may be considered as parasites to prokaryotes because replication and expression machinery is diverted from chromosomal DNA and towards plasmid replication and expression). (Stokes, 2011)

As a final addendum, it may be noted that resistance plasmids and other MGEs typically have a mosaic structure (Gillings, 2015). A resistance plasmid, therefore, may encode for multiple resistance. Resistance carrying Tn21 an example of a mosaic MGE, will be describe in further sections below.

2.2. The fixation of resistance

POPULATION GENETIC variation does not necessarily increase along time because opposite processes (*i.e.*, those that increase, and those that decrease variability) may act on it. The introduction of variation (which may include resistance conferring genes) has already been introduced, and in order to understand how resistance genes become predominant in a population, it is useful to understand processes that deplete variation, such as: (*i*) selection, and (*ii*) drift. Selection is the process that tends to result in the differential survival and reproduction of those exhibiting a particular genotype/ phenotype. A related concept is fitness, which refers to a relative measure of survival and/or reproductive success. Bacterial fitness at the population level is quantified in term of the basic reproduction number (R0). R0 is defined as the number of secondary cases produced from one case in a completely susceptible population (in other words, its transmission potential). R0 must be greater than 1 for a successful parasite, although incursions to < 1values may be permissible for short temporal periods. (Genetic) drift, on the other hand, refers to a change in allele frequency through random sampling of populations. A related concept is a population bottleneck, which is a drastic reduction in population size. Selection may only transitorily reduce population size, while drift is continuous and affects all members of the population regardless of their fitness. At least theoretically, evolution under sole influence of selection would be deterministic, while evolution under influence of drift would be stochastic. The fate of resistance mutations would therefore rest largely on the population size in which they occur. The populations involved in microbial infections vary widely from extreme numerousness (billions in the case of most bacteria) to a single cell (as may be the case in some tuberculosis infections). A small population would be heavily affected by drift while a large population would take larger population reduction in order for drift effects to predominate. It is conceivable that processes governed predominantly by drift would be harder to predict. This is a significant challenge in the prediction of resistance fixation among populations. (Martínez, 2014)

Resistance-conferring mutations occurring under high selection (*e.g.,* high environmental antimicrobial levels) tend to have higher fitness costs and are therefore high risk. On the other case in which resistance-conferring mutations occur under conditions not predominantly governed by selection (*e.g.,* low environmental antimicrobial levels), resistance tend to be associated with higher fitness. Thus, resistance emerging in the former case may be more readily reversible than those occurring in the latter (Andersson, 2014). The difficulty in reversing sub-MIC selection, therefore, is a motivation for establishing minimum selective concentrations (MSC), and for encouraging patient adherence to optimal dosage requirements.

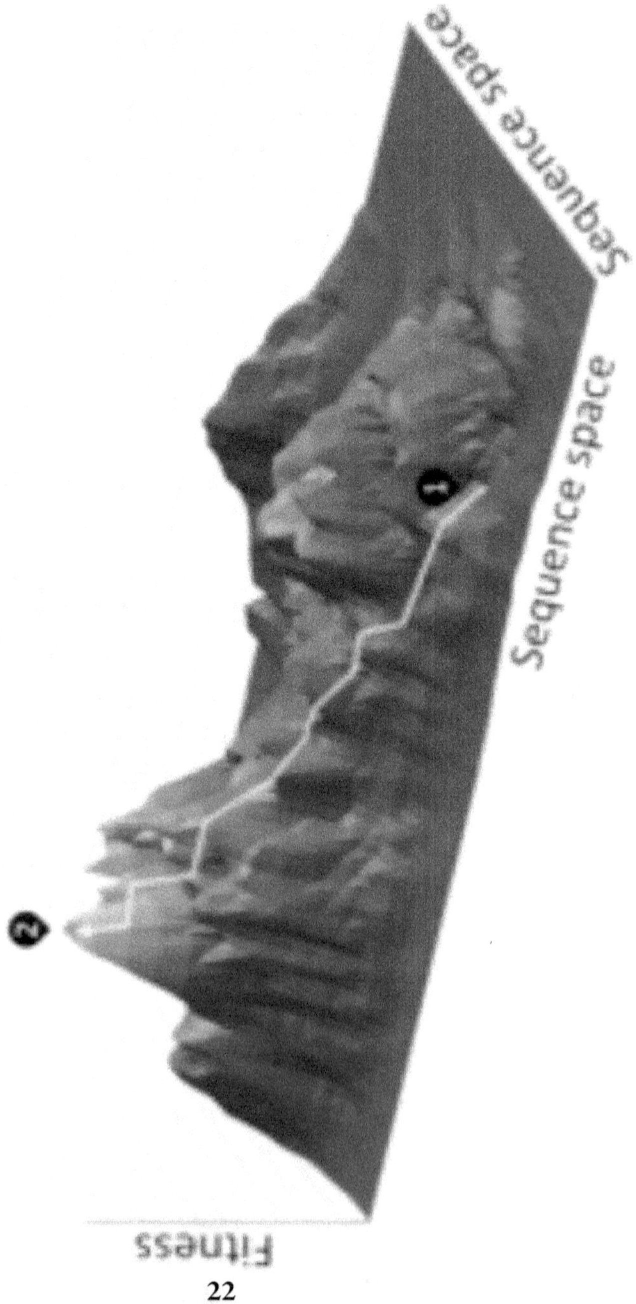
Sequence space
Sequence space
1
2
Fitness

Figure 2. Landscape for multidimensional epistasis. Valkiria Cardoso, CC BY-SA 4.0 <https://creativecommons.org/licenses/by-sa/4.0>, via Wikimedia Commons

3. Anthropologic antimicrobial use

It is now worth looking at the way in which humans have used antimicrobials. Organisms exhibit various types of defense from abiotic and biotic causes of mortality. During much of human evolutionary history the major biotic cause of mortality is infectious disease. Human antimicrobial use has drastically expanded over recent history as a microbial defense strategy in addition to our intrinsic biological defenses. Applying the concept of phenotype extension loosely, human antimicrobial use may thus be considered as an extension of our microbial defense phenotype.

3.1. Historical observations

THE PROBLEM OF ANTIMICROBIAL resistance as a human concern arose with the anthropologic use of antimicrobials. Nevertheless, it is worthy to note at this point that antimicrobial resistance is as ancient as antimicrobial production. For instance, through metagenomics studies, resistance genes have been demonstrated to be present in 'pristine' environments: (*i*) in 30,000 y.o. Beringian permafrost (D'Costa, 2011), (*ii*) in Lechuguilla Cave, New Mexico (Figure 3), in a place that has been isolated for 4M years (Bhullar, 2012), and in 5,000 y.o. Canadian high Arctic permafrost (Perron, 2015). Although there ethnopharmacological evidence of human antimicrobial use dating a couple of thousand years ago, the existence of antimicrobial resistance still greatly predates the relatively recent human antimicrobial use. Anthropogenic antimicrobial pollution, however, has accelerated the emergence, spread, and establishment of resistance.

The existence of the recent antibiotic era has hinged on (*i*) antibiotic drug discovery, and (*ii*) the evolution of resistance (Davies, 2010). Prior to this era, infection management methods have rested largely on hygiene practices and disinfectant use. There was then a golden age of antibiotic discovery during the 1940s and 1950s in which most classes of antibiotics were discovered. A long period of lull soon followed, however, in which the prolongation of the utility of preexisting antibiotics relied on biochemical approaches that involved functional group modification in order to improve target binding and/or pharmacokinetics. Also, the evolution of resistance has managed to catch up with this lagging antimicrobial discovery rate. A recurring fear, therefore, is the approach of a post-antibiotic era in which antibiotics would no longer find utility because it has become more likely that the disease-causing bacteria is already resistant.

During the years surrounding and following the rise of industrial antibiotic production in the 1940s, antibiotics were metaphorically viewed as a 'magic bullet' (Ehrlich) belonging to the human arsenal in a 'war on bugs'. Their use has been directed towards 'anti-biosis' or 'anti-life' of microbes viewed as pathogenic. This classical conception of antibiotics is uninformed by the information that (Landecker, 2015): (*i*) Microbes form communities (biofilm formation) and are engaged in signaling with each other (quorum sensing), and that (*ii*) microbes are able to exchange genetic material (horizontal gene transfer), including those conferring resistance (resistance genes).

At least part of the difficulty in discovering antibiotics is their relatively low concentrations in the environment. Due to the inaccurate conception of antibiotics however, humans have used in great excess (*i.e.*, in lethal levels) of the levels found in nature. This has therefore led to pollution in: (*i*) medical settings (both hospital and community), (*ii*) livestock, agriculture, and aquaculture, and (*iii*) soil and water (Anderssen, 2014). A continuing use of antimicrobials is in animals. Antimicrobials continue to be use for purposes apart from medicine. They are typically used, for example, to increase production yields. In Europe, although strict controls have been set for antimicrobial use in clinical settings, antibiotic sales for veterinary use have continued to increase (Woolhouse, 2015). This double standard in the control of antimicrobials is problematic because the reservoirs of resistant microbes overlap. Although some may be largely confined to humans (e.g., *Acinetobacter*) while some are largely found in animals (*e.g., Salmonella, Campylobacter*), animal-to-human and human-to-animal jumps are well-described in literature (Aarestrup, 2015). For instance, Ward (2014) performed *S. aureus* CC398 discrete trait analysis mapping based on the core genome and inferred ancestral host, and has determined that livestock-to-human jumps have occurred in the span of 30 years. In line with our observation that resistance occurs over various network levels, Ward also noted that mecA (a methicillin resistance gene) transfers have occurred with high frequency.

Metagenomic studies have had great use in describing the effects of antimicrobial use on animal (including human) microbiome (van Schaik, 2015). Anaerobic 'commensals' are major reservoirs for resistance gene. After all, subsequent to antimicrobial use, the entire microbiome is not eradicated and microbes continue to subsist. 'Opportunists' (*e.g., Enterobacteriaceae, Enterococcaceae*), on the other hand, have smaller populations and thus fewer resistance gene transfers. Thus the so-called commensals may play a greater role in conveying resistance than the so-called opportunists. A gap in research is in the role of the host in HGT occurrence in the microbiome. Few studies have been published concerning this aspect. Machado (2014) reported that human intestinal cells modulate HGT. Stecher (2015) noted that gut inflammation increases HGT. Host effects on microbiotal HGT need to be further studied an described.

Apart from the contribution of anthropogenic actions on animals and the environment to resistance, the very social structure of humanity is a factor in resistance emergence. Humans evolved in small, largely egalitarian communities. Larger communities have evolved hierarchy to impose social order. Hierarchies have resulted to greater economic and social inequality. This is a pressing concern particularly in the expansion of society through globalization. It is conceivable that large scale societies have led to large scale inequalities. The gap between developing and developed countries is manifest in their differences in epidemiology. Developing countries, through a combination of various factors (*e.g.,* higher infection incidence & prevalence, inappropriate antimicrobial use) lead to their role as epicenters of resistance genes.

Events that may be cited in support of this observation are: the (*i*) emergence of the New Delhi Metallo- beta-lactamase-1 (NDM-1) that confer resistance to beta-lactam antibiotics, including carbapenems, and (*ii*) the discovery in China of mcr-1 responsible for plasmid-mediated transfer of polymyxin resistance. Further, within individual nation-states, the poor (particularly the urban poor living in conditions promoting high transmission rates) serve as resistance gene reservoirs. The rise of multi drug resistant (MDR)-TB and extremely drug resistant (XDR)-TB has been noted in poverty-stricken communities. These phenomena highlight the shared health of humanity. If antimicrobial resistance is to be addressed, efforts ought to be inclusive.

3.2. A non-anthropocentric view of antimicrobials

THE CLASSICAL CONCEPTION of antibiotics has proven to be inaccurate with additional historical and experiment evidence. In order to avoid errors in research and public health practice, it is important formulate an updated and accurate view of antimicrobials. Most antimicrobials used by humans may simply be part of microbial signal transduction systems, as typically found in nature (Gillings, 2013). For instance, aminoglycosides may be viewed as modulators of 30S ribosomal subunit activity. The same idea may be extended to most antimicrobials and their targets and transporters (*i.e.,* efflux pumps). Evidence to the signaling function of antimicrobials is the observation that antibiotics (at sub-MIC levels) regulate gene expression (Andersson, 2014). Antibiotics like fluoroquinolones, aminoglycosides, and β-lactams (*i*) trigger the SOS response (leading to HGT and recombination events associated with prophage induction, activation of integration and conjugation elements, integron recombination, and transposition), and also (*ii*) trigger RpoS (a stress response sigma factor) induction (leading to increased mutagenesis associated with the action of error-prone polymerases and inhibition of mismatch repair).

The currently known antimicrobials and antimicrobial resistance genes should also be placed in the bigger context of natural reality. Antimicrobials are only a small subset of the microbial parvome (Greek: parvo- small), the set of biologically active molecules. Further, some of the antimicrobials (because only some antimicrobials are peptides) represent a small segment of the panproteome. This means that there is still a wealth of molecules that may be tapped by humans for a variety of microbial management purposes. Also, these small molecules are interacting with numerous proteins that may alter the activity of antimicrobials, or may serve as effectors of antimicrobial function. A description of these interactions would inform antimicrobial use, allowing us to lend subtlety and precision to the ones we utilize. On the other hand, clinically relevant resistance genes are also merely a small subset of the resistome. Gaining understanding of the resistome and the closely associated mobilome may allow us to predict genes with the likelihood of being clinically relevant. Overall, our growing understanding of the microbiome would empower humanity to refine its relationship with our associated microbiota. (Gillings, 2013)

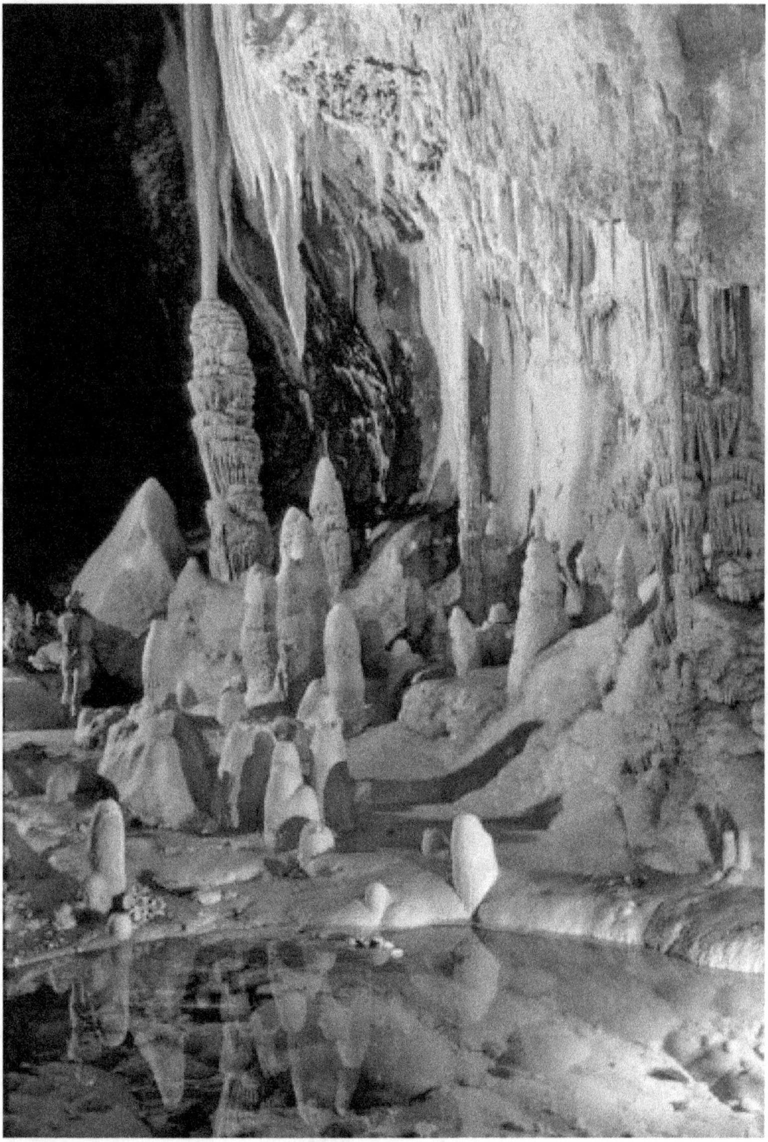

Figure 3. Lechuguilla cave. By Dave Bunnell, CC BY-SA 2.5, https://commons.wikimedia.org/w/index.php?curid=2027473

4. Host-microbe coevolution

4.1. Opposing strategies

Note that the relationship of hosts (*i.e.,* humans) with microbial communities is largely symbiotic, rather than inimical or antagonistic (Méthot, 2014). This is consistent with the predictions of evolutionary game theory that successful strategies would be dominated by reciprocity and generosity. Infectious disease is only one possible outcome of host-microbe interaction. Indeed, microbes associated with infectious disease('pathogens') are a minuscule subset of the global microbiome. Understanding host-microbe interaction, therefore, is core to understanding the motivation behind the human use of antimicrobials (namely to manage infections that afflict us). The traditional approach in defining infectious disease is that it is an outcome of the virulence possessed by a pathogen as an invariant trait. This view is imprecise because it fails to consider the context-dependence of infectious disease. Thus the damage-response framework was proposed by Casadevall and Pirofski (1999) based on the premise that virulence is only a possible outcome of host-microbe interaction. Virulence may have various definitions depending on the perspective, but it may be measured in terms of (*i*) damage resulting from host-microbe interaction, or (*ii*) a decrease in host fitness as a consequence of a microbial infection. Further, recognition of the dependence of infection in its ecological had implications of further infectious disease terminology. For instance, Casadevall and Pirofski (2014) have proposed to downplay—or at least recognize the limitations of—the use of the term 'pathogen' because the ability to cause virulence hinges on the ecological context and there is no exclusive phenotype that delineates pathogens from those that are non-pathogens.

Coevolution is the process involving reciprocal exertion of selection pressures between at least 2 species. Humans and microbes have co-evolved. Indeed, the biggest group of organisms affecting our health is our microbiome. Coevolution involving exertion of adversely selective pressures is termed antagonistic coevolution. According to the Red Queen hypothesis (Valen, 1973; Red Queen refers to the character—in Lewis Carroll's novel Through the Looking-Glass, and What Alice Found There—who made the complaint: Now, here, you see, it takes all the running you can do, to keep in the same place, Figure 4), evolution does not only occur to maximize reproductive advantage, but also to simply survive against competing co- evolving organisms.

When the asymmetric strategies of microbes and humans are taken side-by-side, evolutionary game theory may provide insights. The study of the evolution of cooperation (as pioneered by Robert Axelrod, et al.) finds utility in game scenarios such as the prisoner's dilemma. In a single instance of such a scenario, the best strategy is to defect. Nevertheless, over several iterations, the best strategy is tit for tat (i.e., mimicking the previous move of the opponent). When a further layer of complexity is added to simulations, such as when strategies are made to simulate evolution (*i.e.,* by allowing it to exhibit 'variation' as when multiple strategies are present at the beginning of a simulation, by allowing it to be 'inherited' as when outcome strategies are allowed to be learned over several iterations of the game, and by allowing it to be 'selected' as when more successful strategies are allowed to be iterated in more instances), the strategy that survives is generous tit for tat (*i.e.,* tit for tat that occasionally forgives the betrayal of the opponent). Intuitively, generous tit for tat is better because it precludes destructive cycles in which both players are engaged in minimizing the benefit to each other). A game theory scenario that also finds utility in antimicrobial resistance (especially considering the production of an antimicrobial resistance enzyme in amicrobial population) is the snowdrifter's scenario. The snowdrifter's scenario considers situations involving public goods, such as compounds that benefit not only the producer (*e.g.,* siderophores).

There are as many possible outcomes of host-microbe relationships as there are variations of hosts and microbes. A small fraction of the diverse human microbiota has turned out to exhibit virulence (i.e., a decline in host fitness as a result of infection). In turn, humans respond with its defenses. In other words, human-microbe coevolution may manifest as host-parasite coevolution. Host-parasite coevolution is a form of antagonistic coevolution. In connection with the Red Queen hypothesis, humans and parasites co-evolve for survival. Humans and parasites are involved in an evolutionary arms race, an evolutionary struggle in which adaptations and counter-adaptations escalate over time (*e.g.,* in predator- prey, and host-parasite relationships). In order to illustrate, consider a particular instance of host-parasite coevolution: parasites evolved virulence factors while hosts evolved immune defenses. Over time, the apparatuses and mechanisms involved on both sides may grow in complexity but may have not necessarily pushed the frontlines closer towards a particular side (*i.e.,* driven the extinction of an organism).

If evolution is conceived to be a game involving various trade-offs (*i.e.,* a natural game analogy), a strategy is the set of attributes and behaviors, while fitness would be the payoff. 'Evolutionary strategy' is a metaphor that helps to describe the functional significance of adaptations (Gluckman, 2015). Note that host-parasite coevolution is asymmetric coevolution, in the sense that the strategy of one side is different from that of the other. Microbial strategy for fitness largely involves its (*i*) simple genomics, (*ii*) short generation time, and (*iii*) large population size. In contrast to microbes, a 1% fluctuation in human population may be considered a catastrophe. Human strategy compensates for relatively longer human generation time by having biological complexity, as manifested in the immune and repair systems. The use of antimicrobial agents by humans is an extension of the human antimicrobial phenotype. Life history refers to the entire set of stereotypical patterns characterizing a particular clade. The life history strategy of a particular species is directed towards optimal resource allocation towards maximal reproductive success. Humans and microbes have different life history strategies. One of the many possible trade-offs that may be examined is that between the number versus quality of offspring. The r/K-selection model states that selection pressures drive evolution into 2 general directions: (*i*) r-selection, and (*ii*) K-selection. Microbes are typically r-strategists, i.e., they have shorter generation time, they produce numerous offspring (they have high fecundity) with relatively less longevity, they have small body size, and their population pattern may be described as opportunistic because they typically exploit low-density ecological niches. In contrast, humans are K-strategists, i.e., we have longer generation time, we produce few offspring (they have low fecundity) with relatively greater longevity, we have large body size, and our population pattern may be described to be in equilibrium because our population remain typically close to the carrying capacity.

Antimicrobial use may also be examined through the lens of maladaptive environments. The basic premise of this perspective is that human biology evolved in an environment that is different from the current one, such that traits that had been beneficial has become detrimental. Modern human biology evolved under conditions in which the typical size of social groups is ~150 individuals. Widespread changes in human social organization is associated with a series of demographic and socio-economic transitions with accompanying epidemiologic transitions. The development of human cognition and language has facilitated the growth in complexity of our social structure. Nomadic foraging societies may be considered to be a baseline because ~99.995% of human evolutionary history occurred in these social organizations. Two to three epidemiologic transitions have occurred since then:

a. The first transition occurred with the advent of agrarian societies.,

b. The second transition was concomitant with the Industrial Revolution, and

c. A third transition may be currently taking place along with the rise of globalization.

The general trend of recent human society is towards larger and more complex social organization. These transitions are hereby further examined:

a'. Major human infectious diseases may be roughly grouped into two: (*i*) diseases that have low virulence, low human-to-human transmission, and requiring intermediate hosts (older tropical diseases that could have evolved at a time when population density was lower), and (*ii*) diseases that have high virulence, and high human-to-human transmission (newer temperate diseases that could have evolved at a time when population density has increasing along with the development of settlements). This is associated with the microbial trade-off of virulence for transmissibility. A microbe predominantly engaged in pathogenic relationships with humans has to balance virulence with transmission. The microbe may be too virulent such that the host dies too early before transmission happens, and this is especially disadvantageous in a host population with low density,

b'. Major infectious diseases declined with the advent of better hygiene and the increase in vaccination. Nevertheless, infections appear to be making a resurgence in what may be considered to be another transition, and

c'. The dramatic increase in population, coupled with increased human interconnectedness through globalization, may have led to increased ease in transmission of microbes.

The rise of virulent microbes may be seen therefore to be a consequence, at least in part, of the increase in size of human social groups.

In the human historical time frame, antimicrobial use is ancient. Nevertheless, it is likely that in an evolutionary time frame, antimicrobial use is too recent to have any significant (human)gene-culture co- evolution. Human antimicrobial use may be conceived to be a behavioral/cultural manifestation of our defensive strategies versus biotic (viz., microbial) sources of mortality. Much like the spread of other human technologies, the transmission of antimicrobial knowledge is through cultural transmission. With the transition of human collective learning from less efficient forms (e.g., predominantly vertical transmission of ethnopharmacological knowledge through oral history) to organized study (e.g., academic and scientific efforts towards antimicrobial knowledge acquisition), cultural transmission has increasingly become horizontal.

4.2. The history of host-microbe coexistence

AS MENTIONED BEFORE, host-microbe interactions leading to virulence represent a small segment of the host-microbe interactome. It is therefore important to consider amicable host-microbe relationships (i.e., host- microbe interaction in the microbiome). The history of the microbiome involves changes in selection pressure and diversity over time (Gillings, 2013).

For much of evolutionary history, the primary evolutionary driver of the microbiome was diet, because microbes must be able to persist in the gut with our food as their nutritio. With its discovery, fire then became an important factor because much of the microbes in the diet would be culled by the heat. In the Neolithic, ~11,000 years before present, farming and animal husbandry became important drivers. The microbial diversity of diet was further reduced by human reliance on a few types of crop. Also, the close association with domesticated animals meant that zoonotic jumps between humans and associated animals became frequent. A settled lifestyle also meant the occurrence of larger social groups along with its attendant problems (*e.g.*, sewage management). The Industrial Revolution occurred circa the 18th c. causing further decrease in microbiome species diversity because of the increased consumption of mass- produced processed foods. Pollution and heavy metal utilization also increased during this period. Advances in maritime travel, coupled with the ascendancy of European imperialism and colonialism also facilitated globalization and associated mass transfer of materials (including biotic materials such as microbes). (Gillings, 2015)

An interesting case that demonstrates how genetic studies could be linked to history and evolution is the work on the history of the Tn21 transposon. The Tn21 family of transposons is implicated in the global dissemination of resistance, particularly prevalent among Gram-negative microbes. Pre-1900 when mercury became a significant environmental pollutant, in addition to medical use (*e.g.,* in the treatment of syphilis), the mer operon (conferring mercury resistance) became associated with a replicative transposon, facilitating its dissemination. In a separate occurrence, when quaternary ammonium compounds became prevalently used as disinfectants in the early 1930s, a chromosomal class I integron carrying a qacE gene cassette (encoding for resistance against quaternary ammonium compounds) originating from the Betaproteobacteria chromosome became associated with a Tn402-like transposon. This qacE-carying integron-transposon hybrid was fused to the mer-associated transposon. Industrial antibiotic production followed. When sulfonamide use became commonplace in the late 1930s, sul1 (conferring sulfonamide resistance) was inserted to the 3' end of qacE. In the subsequent decades in which various new classes of antibiotics were discovered and used, the integron carried by the Tn21 transposon was able to capture many different gene cassettes conferring resistance to various antibiotics. (Gillings, 2013; Gllings, 2015)

Whittaker states that total species diversity in a landscape (γ diversity, $\alpha \times \beta = \gamma$) is determined by: (i) the mean species diversity in sites or habitats at a more local scale (α diversity) and (*ii*) the differentiation among those habitats (β diversity).

Applied to the human microbiome, α diversity would be equivalent to species diversity in a microbiome, while β diversity would be equivalent to diversity between the microbiome of human individuals. In the history of the microbiome, α diversity has declined following reduction of dietary bacterial load (concomitant with the human discovery of fire and evolution of cooking and hygiene methods) and diet simplification (concomitant with agriculture and animal husbandry). In contrast, β diversity has increased, suggesting a detachment of individual human microbial identity with that of its environment. This has led to a scenario in which each human individual microbiome serves as a genetic trial-and-error reactor that may lead to the genesis of resistance. (Gillings, 2015)

The history of the microbiome demonstrates the long coevolutionary history of humans and microbes. Perhaps we ought to drive the evolution of less virulent microbes, rather than engage in an unwinnable evolutionary arms race. On order to do this, however, one must understand the principles guiding the evolution of virulence. This will be discussed in the next subsection.

4.3. The evolution of virulence

ANOTHER PROCESS THAT antimicrobial use impacts is the evolution of virulence. The principles behind it are worthy of study if the evolutionary consequences of antimicrobial use, or any other medical approach are to be given importance. The trade-off hypothesis explains a major dilemma that goes as follows (Leggett, 2013): Pathogens/parasites decrease parasite fitness to some degree (by redirection of host resources from host reproduction towards parasite reproduction), but the emergence of highly virulent pathogens/parasites (capable of killing or sterilizing the host) is problematic because it goes against the common assumption that low virulence would facilitate pathogen/parasite transmission (because the not-so-sick host may be better able to spread infectious propagules to the environment or to other hosts). Thus, there is a proposed trade-off between reproduction within the host, and rate of transmission.

The virulence/transmission trade-off is apparent in the rough dichotomy between temperate and tropical diseases (Wolfe, 2007). Tropical infectious diseases (e.g., Chagas' disease, African sleeping sickness, cholera, dengue hemorrhagic fever, malaria, leishmaniasis, AIDS) are typically insect vector transmitted, and also usually involve animal reservoirs. These diseases are usually chronic and/or latent in nature. Only partial immunity or no immunity is obtained. In contrast, temperate infectious diseases (*e.g.*, Influenza A, measles, pertussis, syphilis, tetanus, Hep B, tuberculosis) are mostly acute conditions. Also, long-lasting immunity is usually conveyed. Tropical diseases are expected to expand in the future as a result of global warming (because the vectors would be able to survive in gradually warming areas), and the virulence/transmission setpoint of the top diseases are therefore likely to change.

Changes in human social structure also impact virulence. Humans for much of evolutionary history had low population density and a nomadic lifestyle. Infectious diseases at this period were low virulence (in order to facilitate transmission), and required intermediate hosts (*e.g., Aedes* mosquitoes, *Glossina* flies, *Oncomelania* snails). Coinciding with the first epidemiologic transition, there was an increase in population density (e.g., growth of settlement and village/urban life), the rise of agriculture, and the start of animal domestication in the Neolithic age. The emerging infectious diseases at this period had high virulence and zoonotic origin (e.g., tuberculosis). In the third epidemiologic transition, high transmission rates are observed with the advent of air travel, and the emergence of a unified global society. It is therefore to no surprise that emerging infectious diseases are frequently highly virulent viral infections evolving from zoonotic strains (*e.g.,* because of human contact with livestock, or because of wilderness encroachment).

Aside from the evolution of virulence, another relevant area of study is the genetic basis of infection. After all, virulence is tied to infection. At its core, host-parasite coevolutionary dynamics is determined by the host-parasite genetic interaction. There is a genetic basis whether a particular host-parasite interaction would successfully lead to infection. This genetic basis has conventionally been considered in the framework of two models: the (*i*) matching allele model, and the (*ii*) gene-for-gene model. These two models have been proposed to be the poles of a continuum (Agrawal, 2002). The matching alleles model states that a parasite must match host alleles at infection loci, in order to avoid the host immune system (which is a systems built upon a set of self vs. non-self recognition). This model implies a tight host-parasite specificity. This leads to a Red Queen dynamics in which there is an ongoing advantage for rare genotypes because (i) in the parasite perspective, the rarity may preclude recognition by host defenses, while (ii) in the host perspective, the rarity may preclude the presence of matching parasite genotypes (Luijckx, 2013). There is cyclicality because biological units with a common genotype are selected against such that those units with a rare genotype becomes more emergent. when the rare genotype becomes common, it will eventually be disadvantageous too. In other words, genotype frequencies exhibit oscillatory dynamics when there is a high genetic specificity of infection. Also, the success of infection would be determined by host- parasite genotype interaction, such that only a certain subset of parasite genotype would be infective, while only a certain subset of host genotype is capable of being infected. This model has generally greater appeal in invertebrate zoology. The gene-for-gene model states that successful parasite infection is a result of the interaction between the parasite virulence loci and the host resistance loci. This implies a broad host range for a single parasite genotype. This leads to an arms race dynamics in which a parasite has a set of virulence/avirulence genes while the host has a set of susceptibility/resistance genes, such that in the course of coevolution the host and parasite genes would reciprocally evolve and counter evolve at various loci. Under this model, the success of infection is largely determined by parasite virulence or host resistance, thus parasites possessing virulent genotypes would sweep through the majority of the host population. This may lead to a Suicide King dynamic in which the parasite and/or host is driven to extinction. The general trend implied by this models is that (in the absence of course of infectivity and/or resistance) parasites become super-generalists while hosts become super-resistant. This model has generally greater appeal in plant biology.

Based on the discussion of the previous sections, the parasite population may be seen to have an evolutionary advantage over us humans (the host population), thus facilitating their rapid adaptation to changes in local coevolving humans. Thus, engaging microbes in evolutionary arms races may be inevitably doomed to our failure. The alternative approach presented by a deeper understanding of host-microbe coevolution is to guide the evolution of microbes away from interactions that lead to host damage (*i.e.,* virulence).

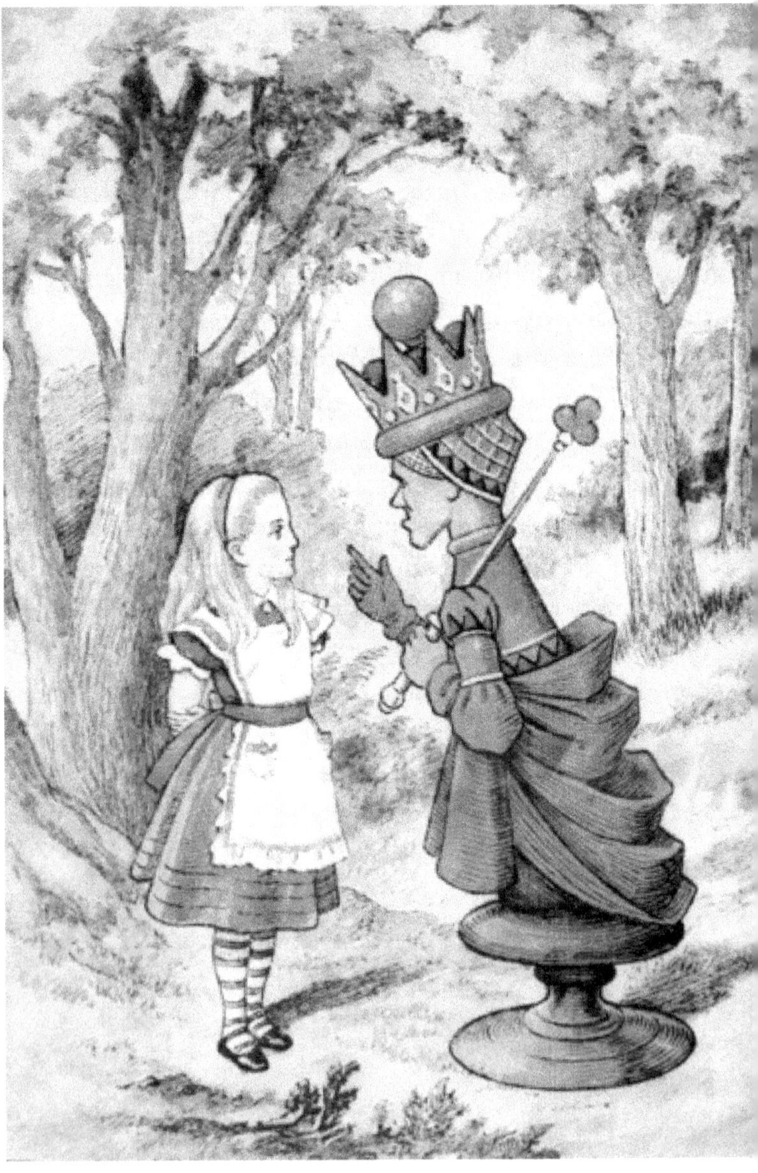

Figure 4. Illustration by John Tenniel of the Red Queen lecturing Alice for Lewis Carroll's "Through The Looking Glass". John Tenniel, Public domain, via Wikimedia Commons

5. Futures

A desirable future scenario is hoped to be achieved by obtaining a more profound understanding of the processes affecting resistance and virulence. Recurring lessons from both historical and experimental evidence is summed up in this section into these two suggestions: (*i*) recognize 'ill' networks, and (*ii*) recognize the evolutionary consequences of humanity.

5.1. Recognize 'ill' networks

RESISTANCE DEMONSTRATE that networks could be 'ill' as well. Increasingly, with the rise of systems approaches in solving human problems, it is being realized that it is not only self-contained units (*e.g.,* individuals) that get sick, but systems and networks could be dysfunctional and generate damaging and destructive outcomes, and therefore be 'ill' as well. In considering virulence and resistance genes, therefore, a GxGxE model is desirable so that these genes are realized to be products of overlaps between host and parasite genotype and phenotype, and their larger environmental context (Méthot, 2014).

Resistance is a multilevel 'ill' network/system. There is an epidemic of resistance genes and MGEs in plasmids. There is an epidemic of resistance-conferring plasmids in bacteria. There is an epidemic of resistant bacteria in the environment. Processes that address these issues would therefore have to work on its different levels as well. (Landecker, 2015)

Baquéro (2008) identified 4 major genetic resistance reactors in which resistance conferring genes are encountered by microbes typically considered 'pathogenic' to humans: (*i*) Animal intestinal microbiota, (especially human and livestock microbiota), (*ii*) locales with high rates of infectious agent transmission, (especially hospitals, with particular regard to maternity and neonatal wards, and intensive care units), (*iii*) areas with high effluent influx (especially sewage treatment facilities), and (*iv*) soil, and surface and groundwater. These, therefore are areas to be targeted by surveillance or remediation efforts.

Efforts have also been made to integrate the cause of human health with the health of the planet as a whole. For instance, one health is the integrative effort of multiple disciplines working locally, nationally, and globally to attain optimal health for people, animals, and the environment (American Veterinary Association, 2016).

5.2. Recognize evolutionary consequences of human action

HOMO SAPIENS has been suggested to be the greatest evolutionary force in the planet (Palumbi, 2001). In line with this, we ought to recognize the evolutionary impact of: (*i*) antimicrobial production and utilization, (*ii*) vaccination (whose capability as an evolutionary force is well documented, as exemplified by the epitope shift in hepatitis B and pertussis, and the failure of Marek's disease vaccine in chickens because of evolution of increased virulence), (*iii*) medicine in general (as such, evolutionary insights have been started to be incorporated in medical education and practice, an instance of which is the drive towards evolutionary medicine by Ewald, Nesse, et al.), and (*iv*) any human action.

The complexity of human culture (including our capacity for collective learning) may be seen as an extension of human biological complexity (as manifest particularly in the human brain and cognition). It is expected that this strategy will be continued in the future to grasp the workings of virulence and resistance, and to act and mold culture accordingly. A deeper understanding of the microbial diversity behind resistance and virulence emergence ought to be obtained as these are the ingredients of evolutionary processes (Casadevall, 2011). Currently, phylogenetic studies and genome projects focus only on human 'pathogens',

and this may be an insufficient and narrow approach. Also, there is a profound connection between human and animal health because the majority of main human infectious diseases transitioned from exclusively animal-infecting towards exclusively human-infecting (Wolfe, 2007). Thus, surveillance of infectious agents should also be performed in animals, at least in those closely associated with humans (*e.g.*, livestock, animals associated with hunter populations). Global harmonization of antimicrobial resistance surveillance (Johnson, 2015) may have utility in keeping track of the various reservoirs (Aarestrup, 2015). There is a wealth in literature describing the evolutionary effects of antimicrobials. Mitchell (2015) reports that antibiotic use may provide pressure that promote the emergence of vaccine escape. Kunkel, et al. (2015) notes that the population-level effects of prophylactic antimicrobial therapy ought to be understood because such preventive strategies may increase, decrease, or have non-monotonic effects on the prevalence of antimicrobial resistance. These are just some examples of the number and variety of published papers allowing awareness of evolution to inform resistance research.

Evolutionary insights could also inform public health interventions (Baquéro, 2015). Efforts may try to: (*i*) Select for susceptible populations, (*ii*) establish susceptible microbiota, (*iii*) reduce HGT of resistance, or (*iv*) decontaminate resistance gene pollution. An example of such evolutionarily informed effort is selection inversion, in which substances interacting with antimicrobials are envisioned to generate inversion scenarios (that select for susceptible strains) as a prelude to subsequent antimicrobial action.

Antimicrobial alternatives are being envisioned and developed, namely (Czaplewski, 2016): (*i*) vaccines, (*ii*) phage therapy (*e.g.*, phage therapy for S. typhimurium in poultry and pigs (Allen, 2013)), (*iii*) synbiotics which are prebiotic-probiotic combinations that may work by generating competition against resistant microbes, (*iv*) predatory bacteria (*e.g., Bdellovibrio bacteriovorus, Micavibrio aeruginosavorus* (Sockett, 2004), (*v*) gene-editing systems (*e.g.*, CRISPR-Cas9), and even (*vi*) metals (*e.g.*, metal-carrying nanoparticles, gallium). Nevertheless, these alternatives are not devoid of evolutionary consequences. Thus, their effects on the future have to be predicted and addressed as well.

As a final lesson from evolutionary game theory, cooperation has evolved and proliferated in populations in which there are mechanisms for the control of cheaters/freeloaders/extortionists that act selfishly in response to the generous actions (*e.g.,* production of public goods) by others. We ought to avoid a tragedy of the commons scenario (Figure 5) in which all utility has been sapped out of antimicrobials because the global society, in effect, has been dominated by cheaters that have not exhibited reciprocal altruism (*i.e.,* have not practiced the attendant responsibilities of antimicrobial use) towards fellow humans.

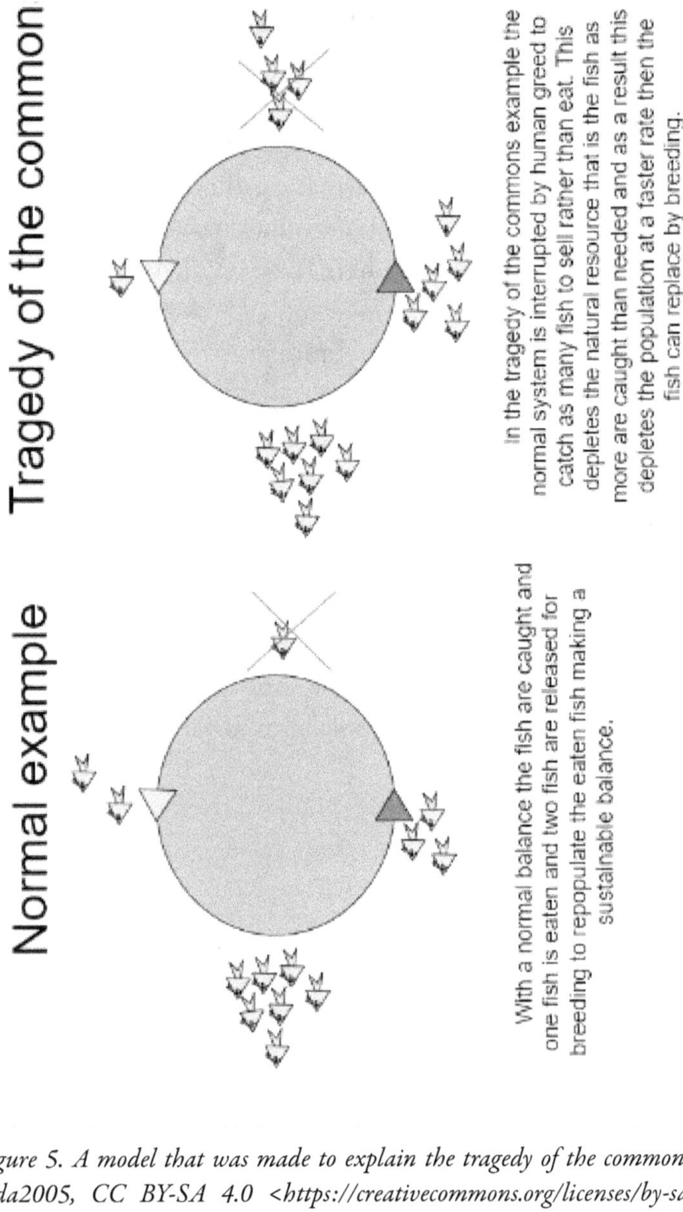

Figure 5. A model that was made to explain the tragedy of the commons. Almeida2005, CC BY-SA 4.0 <https://creativecommons.org/licenses/by-sa/4.0>, via Wikimedia Commons

Concluding remarks

Antimicrobials have extended the microbial defense phenotype of humans. Nevertheless, resistance inevitably arises when antimicrobials are geared towards anti-biosis. Antimicrobials generate evolutionary pressure, to which microbes have the resilient capacity for adapting. Therefore, new efforts ought to focus on ways to drive host-microbe coevolution away from interactions that lead to virulence.

References

General references

American Academy of Microbiology (2010). Antibiotic resistance: an ecological perspective on an old problem. USA: AMA.

Barrett and Armelagos (2013). An Unnatural History of Emerging Infections. Oxford University Press, 93- 108.

Gluckman, P., Beedle, A., and Hanson, M. (2015). Principles of Evolutionary Medicine. UK: OxfordUniversity Press.

Lederberg (1998). Emerging Infections: An Evolutionary Perspective. Emerging Infectious Diseases, 4(3). Mahy, B., ed. (2010). Antimicrobial resistance: Beyond the breakpoint, vol. 6. Switzerland: Karger.

National Academy of Sciences (2010). Antibiotic resistance: Implications for global health and novel intervention strategies. The National Academies Press.

Tibayrenc, M., ed. (2011). Genetics and Evolution of Infectious Diseases, 1st ed. Amsterdam: Elsevier. A gene-based definition of resistance

Allen, et al. (2010). Call of the wild: antibiotic resistance genes in natural environment. Nature.

Blair, et al. (2015) Molecular mechanisms of antibiotic resistance. Nature Reviews Microbiology. doi:10.1038/nrmicro3380

Floyd, J. L., et al (2010). LmrS is a multidrug efflux pump of the major facilitator superfamily fromStaphylococcus aureus. Antimicrob. Agents Chemother. 54, 5406–5412.

Kim, C. et al. (2013). The mechanism of heterogeneous β-lactam resistance in MRSA: key role of the stringent stress response. PLoS ONE 8, e82814.

Kojima, S. & Nikaido, H. (2013). Permeation rates of penicillins indicate that Escherichia coli porins function principally as nonspecific channels. Proc. Natl Acad. Sci. USA 110, E2629–E2634.

Liu, A. et al. (2010). Antibiotic sensitivity profiles determined with an Escherichia coli gene knockout collection: generating an antibiotic bar code. Antimicrob. Agents Chemother. 54, 1393–1403.

Martínez, J.L., Coque, T.M., and Baquero, F. (2014). What is a resistance gene? Ranking risk in resistomes. Nature Reviews Microbiology. doi:10.1038/nrmicro3399

Piddock, L.J. (2006). Multidrug-resistance efflux pumps—not just for resistance. Nature Rev. Microbiol. 4, 629–636.

Tran, Q. T., et al. (2013). The translocation kinetics of antibiotics through porin OmpC: insights from structure-based solvation mapping using Water Map. Proteins, 81, 291–299.

The dwindling antimicrobial drug discovery pipeline

COATES, A.R.M., ET al. (2011). Novel classes of antibiotics or more of the same? British Journal of Pharmacology, doi:10.1111/j.1476-5381.2011.01250.x

Understanding infection as the motivation for human antimicrobial usage

Casadevall, A. and Pirofski, L.A. (1999). Host-Pathogen Interactions: Redefining the Basic Concepts of Virulence and Pathogenicity. Infection and Immunity, 67 (8), 3703-3713.

Méthot, P., and Alizon, S. (2014). What is a pathogen? Toward a process view of host-parasite interactions. Virulence, 5(8), 775-785.

Pirofski, L. A. and Casadevall, A. (2012). Q&A: What is a pathogen? A question that begs the point. BMCBiol. 10, 6.

Pirofski, L. A. and Casadevall, A. (2014). Ditch the term pathogen. Nature, 516, 165-166. Origin of resistance genes

Jansen, A., et al. (2012). Unstable Microsatellite Repeats Facilitate Rapid Evolution of Coding and Regulatory Sequences. Genome Dyn. 7, 108–125.

Shakya, T., and Wrigh, G. (2010). Nucleotide selectivity of antibiotic kinase. Antimicrob. Agents Chemother. 54, 1909-1913.

Stepanova, M., et al. (2008). Convergent in vivo and in vitro selection of ceftazidime resistance mutations at position 167 of CTX M-3 β-lactamase in hypermutable Escherichia coli strains. Antimicrob. Agents Chemother. 52, 1297-1301.

Transmission of resistance

ANDERSSON, D.I. & HUGHES, D. (2014). Microbiological effects of sublethal levels of antibiotics. Nature Reviews Microbiology,12, 465–478. doi:10.1038/nrmicro3270

Gillings, M.R. (2014). Integrons: Past, Present, and Future. Microbiology and Molecular Biology Reviews, 78(2), 257-277.

Norman, A., et al. (2009). Conjugative plasmids: vessels of the communal gene pool. Philosophical Transactions of the Royal Society B. doi: 10.1098/rstb.2009.0037

Soucy, S.M., et al. (2015). Horizontal gene transfer: building the web of life. Nature.

Stokes, H.W., and Gillings, M.R. (2011). Gene flow, mobile genetic elements and the recruitment of antibiotic resistance genes into Gram-negative pathogens. FEMS Microbiology Reviews. doi: http://dx.doi.org/10.1111/j.1574-6976.2011.00273.x

Wozniak, A. et al. (2012). Porin alterations present in non-carbapenemase-producing Enterobacteriaceaewith high and intermediate levels of carbapenem resistance in Chile. J. Med. Microbiol. 61, 1270–1279

The human gut resistome

BUELOW, E. ET AL. (2014). Effects of selective digestive decontamination (SDD) on the gut resistome. J. Antimicrob. Chemother. 69, 2215–2223. doi:10.1093/jac/dku092

Gillings, M.R., Paulsen, I.T., and Tetu, S.G. (2015). Ecology and Evolution of the Human Microbiota: Fire, Farming and Antibiotics. Genes. doi: 10.3390/genes6030841

Machado. A.M.D., and Sommer, M.O.A. (2014). Human intestinal cells modulate conjugational transfer of multidrug resistance plasmids between clinical Escherichia coli isolates. PLoS ONE9. doi:10.1371/journal.pone.0100739

Stecher, B. et al. (2012). Gut inflammation can boost horizontal gene transfer between pathogenic and commensal Enterobacteriaceae. Proc. Natl Acad. Sci. USA 109, 1269–1274. doi:10.1073/pnas.1113246109

van Schaik, W. (2015). The human gut resistome. Philosophical Transactions of the Royal Society B, 370: 20140087. http://dx.doi.org/10.1098/rstb.2014.0087

The natural origin of antibiotic resistance

BHULLAR, K. ET AL. (2012). Antibiotic resistance is prevalent in an isolated cave microbiome. PLoS ONE7, e34953

D'Costa, V. M. et al. (2011). Antibiotic resistance is ancient. Nature 477, 457–461

Perron, G.G., et al. (2015). Functional Characterization of Bacteria Isolated from Ancient Arctic Soil Exposes Diverse Resistance Mechanisms to Modern Antibiotics. PLoS ONE 10(3):e0069533. doi:10.1371/journal.pone.0069533

Evolution of virulence

HALL, M.D., AND EBERT, D. (2011). The genetics of infectious disease susceptibility: has the evidence for epistasis been overestimated? BMC Biology. doi: 10.1186/1741-7007-11-79

Leggett, H.C., et al. (2013). Generalism and the evolution of parasite virulence. Trends in Ecology and Evolution. doi:10.1016/j.tree.2013.07.002

Wolfe, et al. (2007). Origin of major infectious diseases. Nature. doi:10.1038/nature05775 Host-parasite coevolution

Agrawal, A., and Lively, C.M. (2002). Infection genetics: gene-for-gene versus matching alleles models and all points in between. Evolutionary Ecology Research, 4, 79-90.

Chen, P.E., and Shapiro, B.J. (2015). The advent of genome-wide association studies for bacteria. Current Opinion in Microbiology, 25:17-24. doi: 10.1016/j.mib.2015.03.002

Luijckx, P., et al. (2013). A matching allele model explains host resistance to parasites. Current Biology, 23(12), 1085-1088. doi: 10.1016/j.cub.2013.04.064

Ecological perspectives on antimicrobial resistance

WOOLHOUSE, M., ET AL. (2014). Antimicrobial resistance in humans, livestock and the wider environment. Philosophical Transactions of the Royal Society B, 370: 20140083. http://dx.doi.org/10.1098/rstb.2014.0083

Ward, M., et al. (2014). Time-scaled evolutionary analysis of the transmission and antibiotic resistance dynamics of Staphylococcus aureus CC398. Appl. Environ. Microbiol. 80, 7275–7282. doi:10.1128/AEM.01777-14

Multidisciplinary perspectives on combating antimicrobial resistance

AARESTRUP, F.M. (2015). The livestock reservoir for antimicrobial resistance: a personal view on changing patterns of risks, effects of interventions and the way forward. Philosophical Transactions of the Royal Society B, 370: 20140085. http://dx.doi.org/10.1098/rstb.2014.0085

Allen H.K., et al. (2013). Treatment, promotion, commotion: antibiotic alternatives in food-producing animals. Trends Microbiol. 21, 114–119. doi:10.1016/j.tim.2012.11.001

Johnson, A.P. (2015). Surveillance of antibiotic resistance. Philosophical Transactions of the Royal Society B, 370: 20140080. http://dx.doi.org/10.1098/rstb.2014.0080

Kunkel A, et al. (2015) How could preventive therapy affect the prevalence of drug resistance? Causes and consequences. Philosophical Transactions of the Royal Society B, 370: 20140306. http://dx.doi.org/10.1098/rstb.2014.0306

Littmann, J. (2015). The ethical significance of antimicrobial resistance. Public Health Ethics, doi:10.1093/phe/phv025

Mitchell, P.K., et al. (2015). Carriage burden, multiple colonization and antibiotic pressure promote emergence of resistant vaccine escape pneumococci. Philosophical Transactions of the Royal Society B, 370: 20140342. http://dx.doi.org/10.1098/rstb.2014.0342

Rollin, B. (2000). Ethics, science, and antimicrobial resistance. Journal of Agricultural and Environmental Ethics, 14: 29–37.

Ward, M. et al. (2014). Time-scaled evolutionary analysis of the transmission and antibiotic resistance dynamics of Staphylococcus aureus CC398. Appl. Environ. Microbiol. 80, 7275–7282. doi:10.1128/AEM.01777-14

Antimicrobial alternatives

CZAPLEWSKI, ET AL. (2016). Alternatives to antibiotics—a pipeline portfolio review. Lancet Infect Dis, doi:http://dx.doi.org/10.1016/ S1473-3099(15)00466-1.

Sander and Joung (2014). CRISPR-Cas systems for editing, regulating and targeting genomes. Nature Biotechnology 32, 347–355.

Sockett and Lambert (2004). Bdellovibrio as therapeutic agents: a predatory renaissance?. Nature Reviews Microbiology 2, 669-675 (August 2004) | doi:10.1038/nrmicro959

Zasloff (2002). Antimicrobial peptides of multicellular organisms. Nature 415, 389- 395, doi:10.1038/415389a

Anthropogenic impact

GILLINGS, M.R. (2013). Evolutionary consequences of antibiotic use for the resistome, mobilome, and microbial pangenome. Frontiers in Microbiology, doi: 10.3389/ fmicb.2013.00004.

Gillings, M.R., and Stokes H.W. (2012). Are humans increasing bacterial evolvability? Trends Ecol Evol. 27(6):346-52. doi: 10.1016/j.tree.2012.02.006.

Landecker, H. (2015). Antibiotic Resistance and the Biology of History. Body and Society.

Palumbi, S.R. (2001) Humans as the world's greatest evolutionary force. Science 293, 1786–1790

Sandiwà Press is an independent publishing house dedicated to works that unite science, culture, and creativity. *Sandiwà*, from the Filipino words *isang diwa* ("one spirit"), embodies the vision of knowledge as a shared human endeavor. Its publications highlight scholarship, storytelling, and cultural depth, with a commitment to producing works that are both intellectually rigorous and accessible to a wider readership.

Brian Pollo is a physician-educator and writer whose works explore the intersections of medicine, science, and the humanities. His academic background in biochemistry, pharmacology, and clinical practice informs his teaching and research, while his passion for history, literature, and Filipino heritage shapes his creative writing. Through his books, he seeks to make complex knowledge accessible, weaving together scholarship, storytelling, and cultural imagination. His works are published under Sandiwà Press.

Don't miss out!

Visit the website below and you can sign up to receive emails whenever Brian Pollo publishes a new book. There's no charge and no obligation.

https://books2read.com/r/B-A-WMDNE-IHOXG

BOOKS 2 READ

Connecting independent readers to independent writers.

Did you love *Resistance Rising: Genetics, Evolution, and the Future of Infectious Diseases*? Then you should read *Currents of Protection* by Brian Pollo!

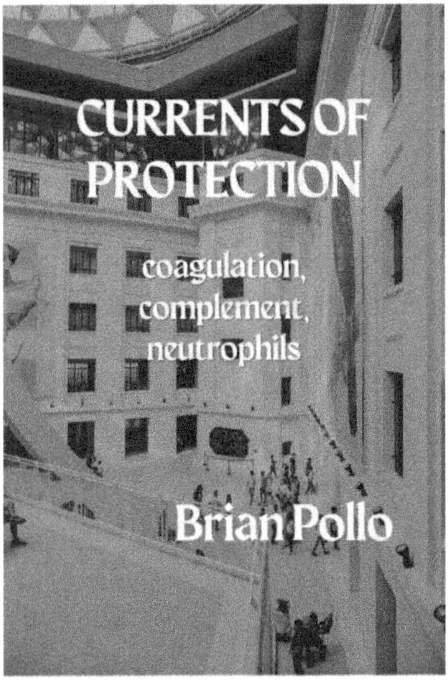

Currents of Protection: Coagulation, Complement, and Neutrophils is a work of creative nonfiction that journeys across science, history, and the humanities to understand the deep entanglement of blood and defense. At its heart is the "triangle" of coagulation, complement, and neutrophils. The three intertwined systems that seal wounds, fight microbes, and sacrifice themselves for the survival of the body. Yet the book insists that this triangle cannot be understood within the laboratory alone. Its story stretches across species, across time, and across the meanings humans have attached to blood.

The opening chapters introduce the triangle of blood and defense, then expand outward into comparative evolution, showing how clotting and immunity appear not only in humans but also in fish, reptiles, birds, and mammals, and even how extremophiles adapt their protective currents to hostile environments. From there, the narrative shifts from biology to history: the blood sciences across time, tracing how ancient physicians, alchemists, and natural philosophers imagined blood's power, and how folk knowledge. The book also reaches deep into prehistory, reconstructing the origins of blood and defense in deep time, then following their arc through human development, from the fetus in the womb to the aged body where protective systems falter. It confronts the darker side of protection, where coagulation, complement, and neutrophils (meant to preserve life) turn against the host, driving autoimmunity, thrombosis, and inflammatory storms. This book contains various chapters on: intervention, where medicine bends these currents through anticoagulants, immunotherapies, and transfusion sciences; semiotics, where symbols, rituals, and metaphors shape cultural understanding; and reconstitution, where gene editing, synthetic biology, and future medicine imagine new forms of protection altogether.

Weaving together molecular biology with anthropology and medical history, *Currents of Protection* invites readers to see blood not only as fluid but as narrative, as system, and as symbol. It is at once a primer on the science of clotting and immunity, a comparative study of defense across the tree of life, and a meditation on what it means to protect and be protected.

For scientists, it offers clarity; for historians, context; for physicians, reflection; for general readers, a story that runs as deeply as blood itself.

Read more at https://sites.google.com/view/brian-pollo/home.

Also by Brian Pollo

Hiyang: Pilipinong Pananaw ng Parmakohenetika
Hiyang: Pilipinong Pananaw ng Parmakohenetika
Salinlunas: Natural Products & Pharmacognosy
Salinlunas: Natural Products & Pharmacognosy
Currents of Protection
Currents of Protection
Resistance Rising: Genetics, Evolution, and the Future of Infectious Diseases
Resistance Rising: Genetics, Evolution, and the Future of Infectious Diseases
Phonies: Authenticity Performance Fakery
Phonies: Authenticity Performance Fakery
Biographies in Blood: The Making of Medical Modernity and Asian Medical Innovations

Watch for more at https://sites.google.com/view/brian-pollo/home.

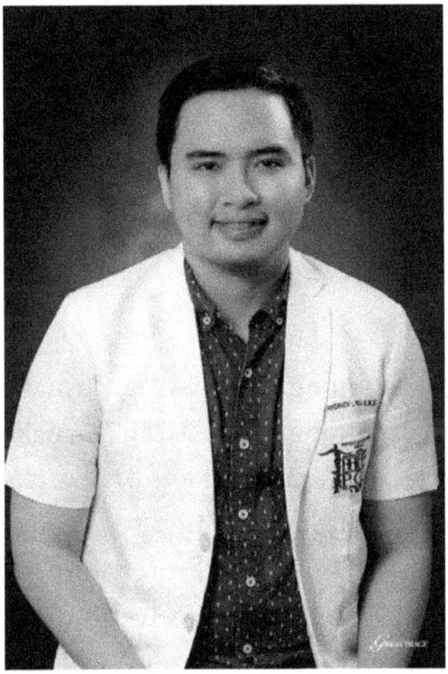

About the Author

Brian Pollo is an MD-PhD candidate, educator, and writer whose work spans biochemistry, ethnomedicine, and the history of science. They study how complement, coagulation, and innate immunity adapt in extreme environments, while also tracing the cultural and symbolic roles of blood in human storytelling. Their writing blends scientific rigor with narrative inquiry, reflecting a commitment to both biomedical innovation and the preservation of ancestral knowledge.

Read more at https://sites.google.com/view/brian-pollo/home.

About the Publisher

Sandiwà Publishing is an independent press devoted to works that unite spirit (*diwà*) and intellect. Its catalogue bridges creative nonfiction, ethnomedicine, history, and the sciences, reflecting the conviction that knowledge is strongest when culture and inquiry walk together. Each publication honors heritage while engaging the challenges of the present, affirming that literature can be both an archive of memory and a spark for new ideas.

Read more at https://sites.google.com/view/brian-pollo/home.

www.ingramcontent.com/pod-product-compliance
Lightning Source LLC
LaVergne TN
LVHW022310200926
848481LV00004B/1267
* 9 7 9 8 2 3 2 7 7 8 4 1 5 *